GUIDE FIVE:
BREAK THE CYCLE

From Root to Tip: A Growing Hands
Guide for Natural Hair

BY CONSTANCE HUNTER

For permissions, inquiries, or additional resources, please contact:

Pre'Vail Natural Hair Salon

www.prevailyournatural.com | prevailyournatural@gmail.com

This book is intended for informational and educational purposes only and should serve as a general guide to understanding and improving natural hair health. While the methods and recommendations provided are based on expertise in natural hair care and trichology, they are not intended to replace professional medical or dermatological advice.

If you are experiencing severe scalp conditions, excessive hair loss, or other persistent issues, it is strongly recommended that you consult a licensed dermatologist or a professional cosmetologist specializing in scalp and hair health. A trained professional can assess underlying causes and provide personalized treatment plans tailored to your specific needs.

By using the information in this book, the reader acknowledges that the author and publisher are not responsible for individual outcomes. Readers should exercise their own discretion when applying the suggested practices.

First Edition: 2025

ISBN:

Paperback: 978-1-968134-05-1

Ebook: 978-1-968134-14-3

Printed in USA

ABOUT THE AUTHOR

As a certified trichologist and natural hair care educator, I specialize in helping individuals discover what's truly possible for their hair—especially when they've been told otherwise.

My passion lies in witnessing transformation—that moment when someone realizes their hair can be healthy, strong, and free. With a deep understanding of the science behind hair and scalp health, I strive to provide clarity, comfort, and actionable solutions. My training equips me to assess and guide care for a wide range of concerns, from common challenges like dandruff and dryness to complex conditions such as alopecia areata, scalp psoriasis, and CCCA.

But my work goes beyond diagnosis or technique. I believe in education, empowerment, and helping clients build routines that nourish their crown from root to tip. This includes learning to read labels, choosing products with purpose, avoiding harmful styling practices, and embracing care that fits their lifestyle and values.

While I offer expert insight from the field of trichology, I'm not a medical doctor. Hair and scalp symptoms can sometimes signal deeper health issues. That's why I encourage a holistic approach—and, when necessary, consulting licensed healthcare professionals for comprehensive support.

In this series, you'll find guidance rooted in science, experience, and care. My hope is that it not only helps you understand your hair better but also love it more, trust it more, and grow with it in ways you never thought possible.

Your hair is not the problem—you just needed the right guide.

DEDICATION

For the one carrying patterns she never chose—
You get to unlearn.
You get to heal.
You get to grow differently.

OVERVIEW

Hair damage doesn't start in your strands—it often starts in your beliefs. *Break the Cycle* is your invitation to unlearn the habits, mindsets, and myths that have kept your hair from reaching its full potential. This guide goes beyond surface-level solutions to address the deeper roots of damage—physical, emotional, and generational.

Whether you're healing from breakage, chemical damage, or years of misinformation, this is your space to reset, rebuild, and grow forward.

SERIES INTRODUCTION

Welcome to *From Root to Tip: A Growing Hands Guide for Natural Hair*

This series was created with one goal in mind: to give you what's been missing—not just products, not just trends, but truth, support, and real guidance for real people who are ready to finally understand and care for their natural hair from the inside out.

For years, we've been taught to manage, fix, or fight our hair. But here, we're doing something different. We're returning to care—not control. To confidence. To consistency. To choice.

Each guide in this series is built as a step in your journey. They can be read in order or on their own, depending on where you are in your process. Whether you're just starting out, rebuilding your relationship with your hair, or deepening your understanding, this space is for you.

I've written these guides from my hands—growing hands that have touched, healed, protected, and restored countless crowns. Now, I offer that care to you.

This isn't just about hair. It's about healing. It's about reclaiming your rhythm, your confidence, and your beauty—from root to tip.

Let's begin.

WHAT YOU WILL LEARN

- How to identify the root causes of common hair damage

- The internalized messages that influence how we treat our hair

- The emotional impact of "fix-it" culture and texturism

- How to shift from control to care in your hair routine

- Techniques to repair damage and build healthier habits

- The truth about trims, transitions, and letting go

WHAT YOU'LL WALK AWAY WITH

- A new, more compassionate approach to hair care

- Tools to interrupt breakage cycles before they start

- Freedom from the myths that keep you stuck

- A renewed sense of trust in your texture, your journey, and yourself

TABLE OF CONTENTS

INTRODUCTION

It's not just about breakage—it's about the beliefs that led to it.

In *Break the Cycle*, we take a closer look at the unspoken rules and outdated practices that have shaped our hair care routines. From hot comb trauma to tight styles to the pressure to conform, many of us have been stuck in cycles we didn't even realize we were in.

But not anymore. This guide shines a light on those patterns—so you can rewrite them. You'll learn how to spot damage early, repair it with intention, and show up for your hair in a way that feels loving, not punishing.

This isn't just repair—it's release.

.

LESSON 1:
DEALING WITH HAIR BREAKAGE

Hair breakage is a common issue faced by many people with naturally textured hair. Understanding the causes of hair breakage and implementing effective prevention strategies can significantly enhance the health and appearance of your hair. This lesson will explore the causes of hair breakage, along with tips for prevention and remedies to strengthen your strands.

Causes of Hair Breakage

Hair breakage occurs when strands become weak and snap off before reaching their full length. Several factors contribute to this issue:

1. Lack of Moisture

Dry hair is more prone to breakage because it lacks the elasticity and flexibility needed to withstand daily wear and tear. Without adequate moisture, the hair cuticle (the outer layer) becomes brittle and susceptible to damage.

2. Over processing

Excessive use of chemical treatments, such as relaxers, dyes, or perms, can weaken the hair's structure. These treatments disrupt the natural balance of the hair, leaving it vulnerable to damage and breakage.

3. Heat Damage

Frequent use of heat styling tools, such as flat irons, curling wands, and blow dryers, can strip the hair of its natural moisture, causing it to become weak and brittle.

High temperatures and a lack of proper heat protection exacerbate the risk of breakage.

4. Physical Damage/ Wet Styling

Rough handling, including vigorous brushing, tight hairstyles, or excessive manipulation, can place physical stress on hair strands, leading to split ends and breakage. Wet hair is particularly fragile and prone to tangling. Detangling wet hair requires patience and the right tools.

Detangling Tips:

- Use a wide-tooth comb or a detangling brush.

- Work in sections and start detangling from the ends, gradually moving upward.

- Finger detangling alone is insufficient as it doesn't remove all daily shed hair.

Styling Suggestion: Consider using low heat when blow-drying to minimize damage, ensuring proper heat protection beforehand.

5. Nutritional Deficiencies

A lack of essential nutrients, such as vitamins and minerals, can negatively affect the health of your hair. Deficiencies in iron, vitamin D, and zinc, in particular, can contribute to weak, brittle strands.

6. Environmental Factors

Exposure to harsh environmental elements such as sun, wind, and pollution can weaken the hair cuticle, leading to breakage. Additionally, swimming in chlorinated water strips the hair of natural oils, causing dryness and damage.

Prevention Strategies

Preventing hair breakage involves adopting healthy hair care practices and making lifestyle adjustments. Below are effective strategies to reduce the risk of breakage:

1. Maintain Proper Moisture Levels

- **Hydrate Regularly:** Use moisturizing shampoos and conditioners tailored to your hair type. Look for products containing hydrating ingredients like glycerin, aloe vera, and natural oils. Avoid products infused with proteins, coconut, or honey if your hair is prone to dryness.

- **Deep Condition:** Incorporate deep conditioning treatments into your routine to provide intense moisture and nourishment. Aim to deep condition at least once a month.

- **Use Leave-In Conditioners:** Apply leave-in conditioners or moisturizing sprays daily to maintain hydration throughout the day.

2. Avoid Over processing

- **Limit Chemical Treatments:** Minimize the use of relaxers, dyes, and perms. If you must use them, follow up with restorative treatments and allow sufficient recovery time between applications.

- **Opt for Gentle Products:** Choose hair products free from harsh chemicals and sulfates to avoid further weakening your hair.

3. Protect from Heat Damage

- **Use Heat Protectants:** Apply a heat protectant spray or serum before using heat styling tools to shield hair from high temperatures.

- **Adjust Heat Settings:** Use the lowest effective heat setting on styling tools. Medium heat on a blow dryer should be the maximum, and it should remain smokeless. For flat irons, use:
  - 400–450°F for coarse, thick hair.
  - 285–325°F for fine, thin hair.

  Apply the "one-pass" method to reduce heat exposure.

- **Limit Heat Exposure:** Decrease the frequency of heat styling. For instance, if flat ironing every two weeks, consider blow-drying and curling instead of straightening.

4. Handle Hair Gently

- **Use Detangle Brush:** Switch to a proper detangling brush instead of wide-tooth combs, as they can cause breakage. Avoid brushes that mimic a spreading hand; these are ineffective.

- **Avoid Tight Hairstyles:** Steer clear of tight hairstyles that put stress on the hair shaft. Opt for loose styles that minimize pulling and tension.

- **Protect Hair While Sleeping:** Use a satin or silk pillowcase to reduce friction, or wear a satin or silk scarf/bonnet to protect your hair overnight.

5. Ensure Adequate Nutrition

- **Balanced Diet:** Eat a nutrient-rich diet that supports hair health. Include foods high in iron, protein, zinc, and omega-3 fatty acids.

- **Hydrate:** Drink plenty of water to promote overall health, blood circulation, and toxin removal. While hydration doesn't directly moisturize hair, it supports the conditions needed for healthy hair growth.

6. Protect from Environmental Factors

- **Wear Hats or Scarves:** Shield your hair from sun and wind exposure with hats or scarves to reduce damage.

- **Rinse After Swimming:** Rinse hair with fresh water before and after swimming to reduce the absorption of chlorine and salt. Avoid using cleansing shampoos immediately after swimming, as the hair is already stripped of natural oils. Instead, replenish moisture with hydrating treatments. The damage isn't from chlorine itself but from its dehydrating effects on hair.

Remedies and Treatments for Strengthening Hair

If your hair is already experiencing breakage, several remedies and treatments can help restore its strength and health. Below are some effective strategies to repair and nourish your hair:

1. Protein Treatments

Protein treatments can strengthen hair strands but should only be used if your hair is not suffering from dryness. These treatments are best applied sparingly.

- **Strengthen Strands:** Protein treatments repair and reinforce the hair's structure. Look for products containing hydrolyzed proteins like keratin, silk, or wheat protein.

- **DIY Protein Masks:** Create homemade protein masks using ingredients such as eggs, yogurt, or avocado. Apply the mask to damp hair, leave it on for 20–30 minutes, then rinse thoroughly.

2. **Moisturizing and Replenishing Treatments**

When damage and breakage are present, correcting moisture levels is essential for recovery.

- **Leave-In Moisturizers:** Use leave-in conditioners and moisturizers to hydrate your hair. Look for products with nourishing ingredients like shea butter, avocado oil, or argan oil.

- **Oils and Serums:** Incorporate natural oils such as jojoba oil or olive oil to seal in moisture and provide essential nutrients.

3. **Scalp Treatments**

A healthy scalp is vital for strong and resilient hair.

- **Scalp Massages:** Regular scalp massages improve blood circulation and promote healthy hair growth. For added benefits, use natural oils like castor oil or rosemary oil during the massage.

- **Exfoliation:** Use gentle scalp exfoliants to remove buildup and dead skin cells. Maintaining a clean and healthy scalp environment can reduce the risk of breakage and encourage hair growth.

4. Regular Trims

Trimming your hair regularly is crucial for preventing further damage and maintaining healthy ends.

- **Prevent Split Ends:** Schedule trims every 6–8 weeks to remove split ends and stop them from traveling up the hair shaft. Regular trims also ease the detangling process. Remember, trimming removes less hair than breakage causes over time.

5. Professional Treatments

For severe breakage or persistent issues, seeking professional help may be the best solution.

- **Consult a Specialist:** A professional stylist or trichologist can provide personalized recommendations and treatments tailored to your hair's specific needs.

By understanding the causes of hair breakage, adopting preventive measures, and using effective remedies, you can improve your hair's health, strength, and appearance. Consistent care and attention to your hair's unique needs will help you maintain strong, vibrant strands and achieve your desired hair goals.

LESSON 2:
ADDRESSING SCALP CONDITIONS

A healthy scalp is fundamental to vibrant, well-nourished hair. Various scalp conditions can disrupt hair growth and overall hair health, making it essential to address these issues effectively. This lesson explores common scalp conditions, their management, and recommended practices for a healthier scalp.

Common Scalp Conditions

1. Dandruff

Dandruff is a common condition marked by flakes of dead skin, often accompanied by itchiness. It is typically caused by an overgrowth of the yeast-like fungus Malassezia, which triggers inflammation and excessive shedding of skin cells.

Management:

- **Anti-Dandruff Shampoos:** Opt for shampoos with active ingredients like zinc pyrithione, ketoconazole, or selenium sulfide to control the fungus and reduce flaking.

- **Regular Cleansing:** Wash your scalp regularly to prevent oil and dead skin buildup.

- **Moisturize:** Use conditioners or treatments to maintain moisture levels and avoid exacerbating dryness.

2. Seborrheic Dermatitis

Seborrheic dermatitis is a chronic inflammatory condition that causes redness, itching, and greasy, flaky patches on the scalp. It shares similarities with dandruff but is often more severe.

Management:

- **Medicated Shampoos:** Use shampoos containing coal tar, ketoconazole, or salicylic acid to reduce inflammation and fungal growth.

- **Avoid Irritants:** Steer clear of hair products with alcohol or harsh chemicals that can worsen symptoms.

- **Hydrate and Nourish:** Apply hydrating conditioners and scalp treatments to maintain moisture and reduce dryness.

3. Psoriasis

Psoriasis is an autoimmune condition characterized by red, scaly patches on the scalp. It results from the immune system triggering rapid skin cell production, leading to the buildup of scales.

Management:

- **Prescription Treatments:** Consult a dermatologist for topical corticosteroids or coal tar solutions to reduce inflammation and slow skin cell turnover.

- **Gentle Cleansing:** Use mild, non-irritating shampoos to avoid aggravating the condition.

- **Moisturize:** Soothe and hydrate the scalp with emollient oils or specialized treatments.

4. Alopecia Areata

Alopecia areata is an autoimmune disorder causing sudden hair loss in small, round patches. It occurs when the immune system attacks hair follicles, often triggered by stress, illness, or other systemic factors.

Management:

- **Topical Treatments:** Use corticosteroid creams or injections to reduce inflammation and stimulate regrowth. In many cases, hair regrowth occurs naturally within 3–4 months.

- **Supportive Care:** Opt for gentle hair care products and avoid harsh treatments that may stress the scalp further.

- **Consult a Specialist:** Seek advice from a dermatologist or trichologist if regrowth hasn't begun after three months.

5. **Itchy Scalp**

An itchy scalp can result from dryness, allergies, or infections. Persistent itching may lead to discomfort, scratching, and scalp damage.

Management:

- **Identify Triggers:** Pinpoint allergens or irritants in your hair care routine and make adjustments accordingly.

- **Soothing Treatments:** Use scalp treatments containing aloe vera, tea tree oil, or sulfur to reduce irritation. Lightly moisturizing the scalp with a suitable product can also help.

- **Avoid Over-Scratching:** Keep nails short and avoid scratching to prevent further irritation and damage.

Recommended Products and Practices for a Healthy Scalp

1. Cleansing Products

- **Mild Shampoos:** Opt for gentle shampoos free from harsh sulfates. Choose products tailored to your specific scalp needs, such as anti-dandruff or moisturizing formulas.

- **Clarifying Shampoos:** Use a clarifying shampoo occasionally to remove product buildup and impurities. Avoid overuse to prevent stripping the scalp of its natural oils.

2. Conditioning Products

- **Hydrating Conditioners:** Select conditioners that provide moisture and nourishment. Ingredients like shea butter, argan oil, and glycerin are particularly effective for maintaining hydration.

- **Scalp Treatments:** Incorporate treatments designed specifically for the scalp to address targeted concerns, such as soothing irritation, exfoliating dead skin, or boosting moisture.

3. Treatment Products

- **Anti-Dandruff Solutions:** Choose treatments with active ingredients like zinc pyrithione, ketoconazole, or selenium sulfide to manage dandruff and seborrheic dermatitis.

- **Moisturizing Oils:** Natural oils like jojoba, argan, or almond oil are excellent for hydrating and soothing the scalp.

- **Medicated Creams:** For conditions like psoriasis or severe dandruff, consult a dermatologist and use medicated creams or solutions as prescribed.

4. Healthy Practices

- **Regular Washing:** Maintain a consistent washing routine to keep your scalp clean and free from excess oil and buildup. Adjust the frequency based on your scalp's specific needs.

- **Gentle Massage:** Incorporate gentle scalp massages into your routine to stimulate blood flow and encourage relaxation. Avoid applying excessive pressure or aggressive rubbing.

- **Avoid Harsh Products:** Avoid hair products containing alcohol, sulfates, or artificial fragrances, as these can irritate the scalp. Choose natural or hypoallergenic products whenever possible.

- **Balanced Diet:** Ensure your diet includes essential nutrients for scalp health, such as vitamins, minerals, and omega-3 fatty acids. A well-balanced diet supports overall skin health and improves scalp condition.

- **Hydration:** Drink plenty of water to maintain overall hydration, which supports both scalp and hair health.

By understanding common scalp concerns and adopting effective management strategies, you can achieve a healthier, more balanced scalp. Using the right products and practices tailored to your scalp's needs will promote optimal hair health and help address any challenges that arise.

LESSON 3:
BUILDING CONFIDENCE AND SELF-ESTEEM

Embracing natural hair can be a profound journey toward self-acceptance and confidence. For many, it represents more than a style choice; it symbolizes a deep connection to identity, culture, and self-worth. This discussion explores how embracing natural hair can enhance confidence and self-esteem, while addressing the challenges posed by societal pressures and fostering self-love.

Embracing Natural Hair as a Source of Confidence

Natural hair serves as a form of personal expression and a reflection of one's heritage and individuality. Choosing to wear hair in its natural state is an empowering decision that reclaims cultural and personal identity. Here's how embracing natural hair can boost confidence and self-esteem:

1. Connection to Identity

Natural hair is often a powerful expression of cultural and personal identity. For individuals of African descent, natural textured hair embodies a connection to ancestral roots and heritage. Celebrating this aspect of one's identity can foster a sense of pride and belonging. Aligning with cultural history and personal identity often translates into higher self-esteem and confidence.

2. Authenticity and Self-Acceptance

Wearing natural hair encourages individuals to embrace their authentic selves. In a world where societal beauty standards often favor straight or chemically altered hair, choosing natural hair is both an act of self-acceptance and a defiance of those norms.

This journey toward authenticity can lead to greater self-acceptance and confidence as individuals learn to value and celebrate their unique qualities.

3. Empowerment Through Self-Care

Caring for and styling natural hair can be an empowering practice. Learning about hair care, experimenting with styles, and developing personalized routines foster a sense of accomplishment and control. Seeing the positive results of these efforts reinforces self-worth and builds confidence.

4. Role Modeling and Representation

By embracing natural hair, individuals become role models and advocates within their communities. Representation matters. Seeing diverse forms of beauty, including natural hair, inspires others to embrace their unique attributes. This positive ripple effect enhances self-esteem, not only for the individual but also for those who look up to them.

Overcoming Societal Pressures and Embracing Self-Love

Despite the personal and cultural significance of natural hair, societal pressures can pose challenges. Navigating these pressures requires addressing external influences while cultivating self-love.

1. Navigating Societal Standards of Beauty

Narrow societal beauty standards often favor specific hair types and textures, creating pressure to conform.

Overcoming these standards involves recognizing and challenging such biases.

Beauty is diverse and subjective, and true self-worth stems from personal acceptance, not societal norms.

2. Dealing with Negative Comments and Criticism

Negative comments about natural hair can be disheartening. Building resilience is key to managing these reactions. Strategies include practicing positive self-talk, seeking support from like-minded individuals, and engaging with communities that celebrate natural hair.

3. Cultivating Self-Love

Self-love is essential for overcoming societal pressures. Nurturing a positive self-image involves affirmations, self-care routines, and engaging in activities that reinforce self-worth. It's important to remember that self-worth is inherent and independent of appearance.

4. Creating a Supportive Environment

A supportive network makes a significant difference in building confidence. Joining communities that celebrate natural hair and diverse beauty standards provides encouragement, shared experiences, and positive reinforcement.

5. Educating and Advocating

Educating others about the beauty and significance of natural hair is a powerful tool for change. Advocacy includes challenging stereotypes, promoting inclusivity, and encouraging a broader understanding of beauty. Participating in these conversations helps foster an inclusive society and highlights the universal challenges of hair care, regardless of texture.

6. Setting Personal Goals

Personal goals related to hair care and self-improvement can provide motivation and purpose. Whether mastering new styling techniques, learning about hair health, or focusing on personal growth, setting clear objectives enhances confidence and provides a sense of accomplishment.

Embracing natural hair as a source of confidence and self-esteem requires a multifaceted approach. Personal acceptance, resilience against societal pressures, and cultivating self-love are key components. By celebrating unique attributes and advocating for more inclusive beauty standards, individuals can build a strong sense of self-worth and confidence.

QUIZ
OVERCOMING CHALLENGES

Lesson 1: Dealing with Hair Breakage

1. Question

Which of the following is a common cause of hair breakage?

a) Over-moisturizing the hair.

b) Low Heat styling without protection.

c) Over use of protein, coconut and honey.

d) Deep conditioning too often.

Answer: C) over use of protein, coconut and honey.

2. Question

Which of the following is a prevention strategy for hair breakage?

a) Regular trimming of split ends.

b) Skipping conditioning treatments.

c) Washing hair daily.

d) Using harsh combs and brushes.

Answer: a) Regular trimming of split ends.

3. Question

What is one of the most effective remedies for strengthening weak, damaged hair?

a) Daily shampooing with a clarifying product.

b) moisture treatments and deep conditioning.

c) Avoiding oil-based treatments.

d) Using Protein treatments.

Answer: b) Moisture treatments and deep conditioning.

Lesson 2: Addressing Scalp Conditions

1. Question

Which of the following is a common scalp condition that can affect hair growth?

a)   Oily scalp.

b)   Dandruff.

c)   Split ends.

d)   Frizzy hair.

Answer: b) Dandruff.

2. Question

Which ingredient is commonly recommended to treat scalp irritation and promote a healthy scalp?

a)   Mineral oil.

b)   Tea tree oil.

c)   Perfume.

d)   Silicones.

Answer: b) Tea tree oil.

3. Question

What is one recommended practice for maintaining scalp health?

a)   Washing the hair only once a month.

b)   Avoiding moisture-based products.

c) Massaging the scalp regularly to increase blood circulation.

d) Only using heat to dry the scalp.

Answer: c) Massaging the scalp regularly to increase blood circulation.

Lesson 3: Building Confidence and Self-Esteem

1. Question

Why is embracing natural hair often seen as a source of confidence?

a) It represents authenticity and self-acceptance.

b) It requires less maintenance than straightened hair.

c) It conforms to beauty standards set by society.

d) It eliminates the need for hair care routines.

Answer: a) It represents authenticity and self-acceptance.

2. Question

Which of the following is an effective way to overcome societal pressures regarding natural hair?

a) Changing your hair to fit societal norms.

b) Embracing self-love and rejecting unrealistic beauty standards.

c) Avoiding public discussions about hair.

d) Using chemical treatments to alter natural hair texture.

Answer: b) Embracing self-love and rejecting unrealistic beauty standards.

3. Question

How can building a supportive community help in overcoming challenges related to natural hair?

a) It provides external validation for changing hair texture.

b) It helps individuals feel empowered and supported in their natural hair journey.

c) It reinforces the need to conform to mainstream beauty standards.

d) It promotes only one type of hairstyle for everyone.

Answer: b) It helps individuals feel empowered and supported in their natural hair journey.

4. Question

What is a significant personal benefit of embracing your natural hair and style?

a) Increased hair growth rate.

b) Higher self-esteem and self-acceptance.

c) Faster hair styling routine.

d) Avoiding the use of hair care products altogether.

Answer: b) Higher self-esteem and self-acceptance.

CLOSING NOTE

You don't have to carry every method, mindset, or
memory.
Some things were never yours to begin with—and now,
you get to let them go.

www.ingramcontent.com/pod-product-compliance
Lightning Source LLC
Chambersburg PA
CBHW052143270326
41930CB00012B/2998